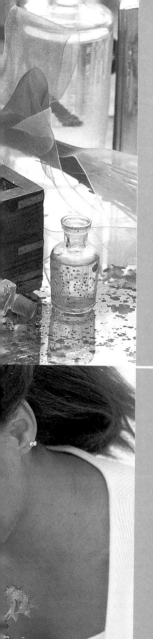

introduction

People have been using scented products since time began in religious ceremonies, in massage, in the bath and for scenting the hair and body. It was not until the 10th century AD, however, that Arabic physicians learned how to distil pure essential oils from plants.

Aromatic plants contain essential oils, which are used to relax, sedate, refresh or stimulate according to need. These essential oils have been found to have significant healing properties, in addition to affecting moods. Nowadays, widespread use is made of aromatherapy in many fields of conventional medicine.

Essential oils

Essential oils are natural, volatile substances that evaporate readily, releasing their aroma into the air, as happens, for example, when someone brushes against an aromatic plant. The oils have many beneficial properties.

A widely used method of employing essential oils in the home is to fragrance the rooms by means of a vaporizer or oil burner. Although vaporizers come in many forms, they all work on the same principle. The reservoir is filled with water, to which are added a few drops of essential oil. The reservoir is then heated, which causes the oil and water to evaporate. The heat must be fairly low to allow slow evaporation of the oil and a longer-lasting scent.

Adding a few drops of essential oil to a bowl of hot water is a pleasant way of adding scent to a room, especially in a dry atmosphere.

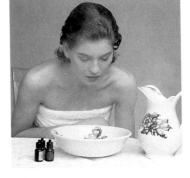

▲ ADD ESSENTIAL OILS TO HOT WATER FOR A BENEFICIAL STEAM INHALATION.

Choose an attractive bowl and place it out of reach of children. Use an oil that you really like, as its fragrance will linger for some time. You can also use the bowl of scented water for an uplifting or calming steam inhalation. Essential oils can be used to make a luxurious addition to the bath, whether they are chosen to aid recovery from an illness, to lift the spirits, or to promote relaxation after a stressful day.

▶ OIL BURNERS CAN MAKE ATTRACTIVE ROOM ORNAMENTS.

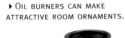

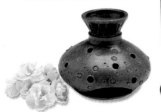

healing with aromatherapy

a concise guide
to using essential oils
for health, harmony
and happiness

HERMES
HOUSE

The edition published by Hermes House

© Anness Publishing Limited 2002 updated 2003..

Hermes House is an imprint of Anness Publishing Limited,
Hermes House, 88–89 Blackfriars Road, London SE1 8HA

Publisher: Joanna Lorenz
Production Controller: Joanna King

Publisher's Note:
The Reader should not regard the recommendations, ideas and techniques
expressed and described in this book as substitutes for the advice of a
qualified medical practitioner or other qualified professional.
Any use to which the recommendations, ideas and techniques
are put is at the reader's sole discretion and risk.

Printed in Hong Kong/China

3 5 7 9 10 8 6 4

contents

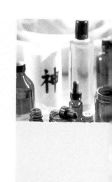

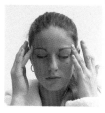

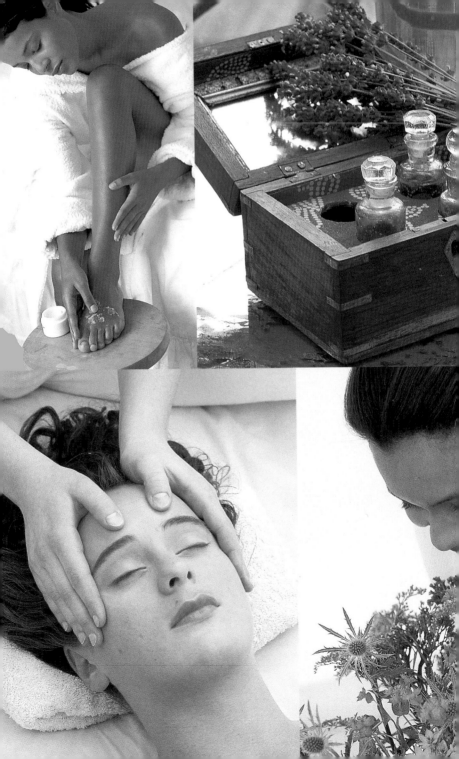

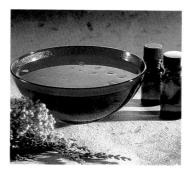

▲ A FEW DROPS OF ESSENTIAL OIL IN HOT WATER WILL PERFUME A ROOM.

The essential oils recommended for the bath affect the body as they are inhaled in the steam, but some also penetrate the skin pores that open in the warmth.

In order to add oils to the bath safely it is important to dilute them in vegetable oil, cream or full-fat milk. Add the blend to the bathwater, just before the bath has filled to the desired depth, pouring it slowly under the hot water tap so the oil disperses through the air and water.

▼ SLOWLY ADD DILUTED OIL TO BATHWATER.

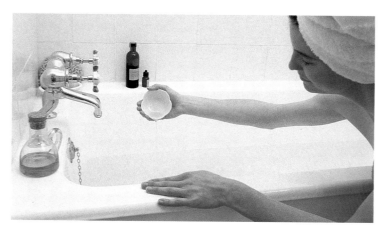

Preparing & storing essential oils

When essential oils are used for aromatherapy massage, different oils are combined to increase their therapeutic effect. Once you have mixed your oils, store and use them immediately, as they are perishable.

Aromatic essential oils may be used in a number of ways to maintain and restore health, and to improve our quality of life with their scents. Essential oils are concentrated substances and as such they need to be diluted for safety and optimum effect.

The ratio of essential oil to carrier oil varies, but as a rule, ten drops of essential oil in 20ml/4 tsp carrier oil is enough for a body massage. This gives a standard 2.5 per cent dilution, recommended for most uses.

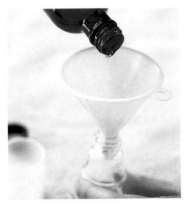

▲ USE A FUNNEL TO AVOID SPILLAGE.

Experiment with different types of vegetable oil to find the ideal blend for your massage style. Add a teaspoonful of another vegetable oil as well as the essential oils for an exotic and personal mixture.

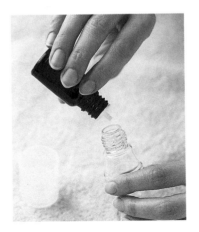

◄ BLEND OILS ONE DROP AT A TIME.

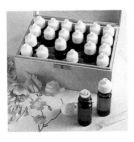

► STORE OILS IN DARK BOTTLES.

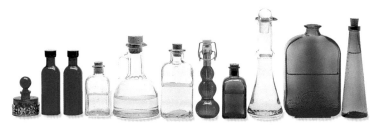

To blend essential oils for massage, first pour the vegetable oil into a blending bowl. Then add the essential oil a drop at a time and mix gently with a cocktail stick to blend. Test the fragrance before beginning the massage; it may require slight adjustment.

Essential oils are liable to deteriorate through the action of sunlight, so should be stored in a cool, dark place and away from direct heat. They should always be bought in dark-coloured glass bottles with a stopper that dispenses them a drop at a time. Only blend a small quantity of oils at a time to prevent the mixture deteriorating. Citrus oils tend to go off more quickly than other oils, so it is best to buy them in small amounts as you need them.

▲ STORE CARRIER OILS CAREFULLY TO ENSURE THEIR FRESHNESS.

▼ USE AROMATHERAPY BLENDS IMMEDIATELY OR STORE IN SEALED BOTTLES AS ESSENTIAL OILS EVAPORATE QUICKLY.

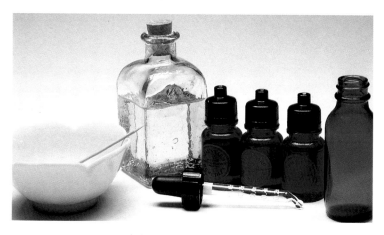

Citrus oils

Many citrus fruits yield essential oils, and they tend to have similar properties. In general they are refreshing, stimulating oils, good for the morning bath, leaving you feeling cleansed and alive.

ORANGES

The bitter, or Seville, orange is the source of three different oils, from the fruit, the blossom (also known as neroli) and the leaf (also called petitgrain). All have a mellow, warming and soothing effect, and are a good tonic and mood lifter, raising the libido.

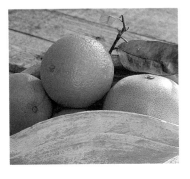

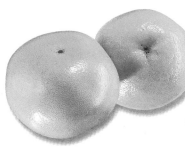

GRAPEFRUIT

This uplifting oil, taken from the fruit's fresh peel, helps to digest fatty foods, and combat cellulite and congested pores. It also soothes headaches and nervous exhaustion.

NEROLI

This oil is particularly effective for nervous tension, headaches, insomnia and other stress-related conditions. It can also be used to create a feeling of peace and is useful during times of anxiety, panic, hysteria or shock and fear. It can also help in the development of self-esteem and self-love.

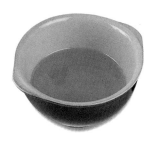

LIMES

Oil of lime is good for stimulating a sluggish system and may be used when a tonic is needed, in massage or in the bath.

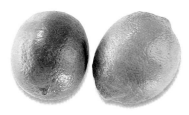

MANDARINS

Refreshing and cleansing, this sweetly scented oil is especially good for skin problems such as acne. It also helps digestion, soothing heartburn and nausea.

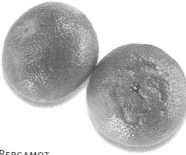

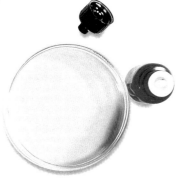

BERGAMOT

The peel of the ripe fruit yields an oil that is mild and gentle. It is the most effective antidepressant oil of all, best used at the start of the day. The oil can be used on a burner for lifting the atmosphere. Do not use on the skin in bright sunlight, as it can cause irritation.

LEMONS

Possibly the most cleansing and antiseptic of the citrus oils, lemon oil is useful for boosting the immune and respiratory systems, and for use in skin care. It can also refresh and clarify thoughts, preventing feelings of bitterness or resentment about life's injustices.

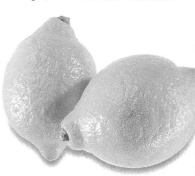

Shrub & vine oils

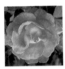

Essential oils can be extracted from many different parts of plants. Rose and jasmine oils are obtained from the flowers, the oil of black pepper comes from the fruit of a tropical vine, and geranium oil is taken from the plant's leaves.

JASMINE

One of the most wonderful aromas, jasmine has a relaxing, euphoric effect, and can lift the mood when there is debility, depression and listlessness. Use in the bath or in massage oils.

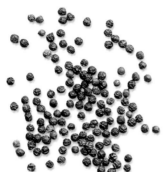

BLACK PEPPER

The essential oil of black pepper is warming and comforting and can often add mysterious depth to a blend. Black pepper is particularly effective for muscular aches and pains, colds and fevers.

GERANIUM

Rose-scented geranium oil is obtained from the shrub's leaves. It has a refreshing antidepressant quality, which is good for nervous tension and exhaustion, and can combine a blend to make a more harmonious scent.

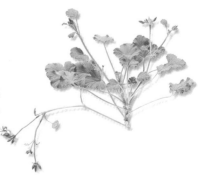

Lavender

Extracted from lavender flowers, this oil is the most versatile of all essential oils. It has been used for centuries to refresh and add fragrance to the home, and as a remedy for stress-related ailments.

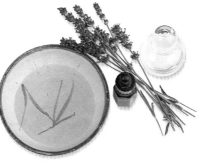

Juniper

Good for strengthening the spirits and purifying the atmosphere, this oil is obtained from juniper berries. Its most important use is as a detoxifier, but it is also effective for cystitis, cellulite, water retention, and absence of or painful menstrual periods.

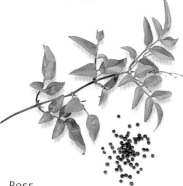

Rose

Probably the most famous of all oils, rose is good for sedating, calming and as an effective anti-inflammatory. Use in the bath or add to a base massage oil to soothe muscular and nervous tension.

Rosemary

This stimulating oil, taken from the plant's leaves, has been used for centuries to help relieve nervous exhaustion, tension headaches and migraines. It improves circulation to the brain, and is an excellent oil for mental fatigue and debility. It is also an effective remedy for fluid retention.

Herb & spice oils

The essential oils of many herbs and spices contain powerful healing properties, which should be enjoyed but also respected. Nature provides an abundance of therapeutic compounds to help restore health and vitality.

CLARY SAGE

This essential oil, taken from the leaves, gives a euphoric uplift to the brain; be careful how much you use, however, as it can leave you feeling very intoxicated! Its relaxing and antidepressant qualities have contributed to its reputation as an aphrodisiac.

PEPPERMINT

The plant's leaves are used to produce this oil which is a classic ingredient in inhalations for relieving catarrh. Peppermint's analgesic and antispasmodic effects make it very useful for rubbing onto the temples to ease tension headaches; ideally dilute a drop in a little base cream or oil before applying.

CHAMOMILE

The flowering parts of Roman and German chamomile are used to obtain essential oils with very similar properties. Chamomile oil is relaxing and antispasmodic, and helps to relieve tension headaches, nervous digestive problems and insomnia. It is also a gentle sedative oil for people who are highly strung and over-enthusiastic.

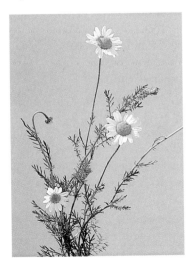

MARJORAM

Obtained from marjoram leaves, this oil has a calming and warming effect, and is good for both cold muscles and for cold and tense people who might also suffer from headaches, migraines or insomnia.

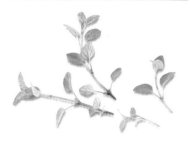

GINGER

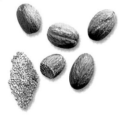

Extracted from the ginger root, this oil is known for its warm and comforting nature. It is a balancing oil and counteracts ailments caused by dampness, being particularly effective for muscular aches and pains, catarrh and other symptoms of coughs and colds.

NUTMEG

Warming, stimulating and euphoric, this oil, taken from the fruit of the nutmeg tree, is good for poor circulation, muscular aches, sluggish digestion, loss of appetite and the early stages of a cold. It can also be comforting to those who feel emotionally isolated.

PALMAROSA

Taken from the leaves of this herbaceous plant, palmarosa is a gentle and comforting oil. It is particularly effective for acne, dermatitis, scars, sores and other skin inflammations, as well as weak digestion, headaches and nervous exhaustion.

Tree oils

Oils can be obtained from a variety of trees; with some, for example, cedarwood, the oil is extracted by steam distillation from the wood, whereas with others, such as ylang ylang, the oils come from the flowers.

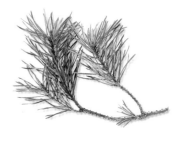

PINE
The pine oil used in aromatherapy generally comes from the Scots pine. It helps to clear the air passages when used as an inhalation, and is also good for relieving fatigue. Tired, aching muscles can be eased with massage using diluted pine oil.

EUCALYPTUS
Extracted from eucalyptus leaves, this is one of the finest oils for respiratory complaints, eucalyptus is found in most commercial inhalants. Well diluted in a base vegetable oil, eucalyptus can be applied to the forehead to help relieve a hot, tense headache linked with tiredness.

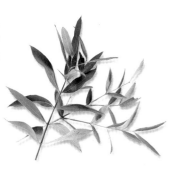

TEA TREE
Vigorous and revitalizing, tea tree oil is effective in fighting infectious organisms. It is also a powerful immune stimulant, increasing the body's ability to respond to these organisms.

SANDALWOOD

Probably the oldest perfume in history, sandalwood has been used for 4,000 years. It has a heavy scent, and often appeals to men as much as to women. It has a relaxing, antidepressant effect on the nervous system, and where depression causes sexual problems, sandalwood can be used as a genuine aphrodisiac.

CEDARWOOD

Thought to be one of the earliest known essential oils, cedarwood oil is effective for long-standing complaints rather than acute ones, such as acne, dandruff, arthritis, rheumatism, bronchitis and chest infections. This uplifting oil is useful for treating lack of confidence or fearfulness, and can help to eliminate mental stagnation. Its relaxing and soothing properties can be a good aid to meditation. Cedarwood is also an aphrodisiac.

CYPRESS

With a rich scent similar to the scent of pine needles, cypress oil is useful for treating conditions that cause excess fluids, such as diarrhoea, water retention and watery colds. The oil, extracted from the tree's cones, can be uplifting in cases of sadness or self-pity, and can help to soothe anger.

YLANG YLANG

The flowers of this tropical tree, native to Indonesia, produce an intensely sweet essential oil that has a sedative yet antidepressant action. It is good for many symptoms of excessive tension, such as insomnia, panic attacks, anxiety and depression.

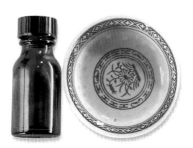

Aromatherapy massage

Massage is a wonderful way to use essential oils, suitably diluted in a good base oil, for your partner or family. Use soft, thick towels to cover areas of the body you are not massaging, and make sure that the room is warm.

Anyone will benefit from regular massage as it eases tense muscles and also helps us feel warm and relaxed. Although quite different and inevitably limited, self-massage is also an excellent way to help yourself relax and can help clear tension headaches and ease a stiff neck and shoulders.

Ideally, massage should be carried out just before a bath or when you can lie down in a warm place. Suitable base oils for massage include sweet almond oil (probably the most versatile and useful), grapeseed, safflower, soya (a bit thicker and stickier), coconut and even sunflower. For very dry skins, a small amount of jojoba, avocado or wheatgerm oils (except in cases of wheat allergy) may be added. Essential

▼ THE NURTURING TOUCH OF MASSAGE IS ENHANCED BY THE AROMA OF ESSENTIAL OILS.

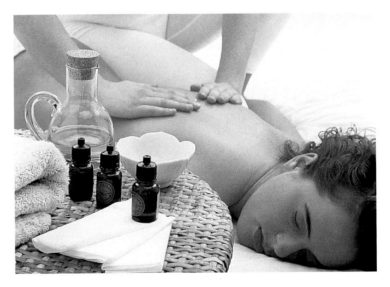

oils may be blended at a dilution of 1 per cent, or one drop per 5ml/1 tsp base oil; this may sometimes by increased to 2 per cent, but take care that no skin reactions occur with any oil.

If someone has sensitive skin or suffers from allergies, try massaging with one drop of essential oil per 20ml/4 tsp base oil to test for any reaction. Seek medical advice before massaging a pregnant woman.

Prepare for massage by playing some soft music, lowering the lights or lighting candles and ensure your partner is lying comfortably on the floor with a clean towel spread beneath them.

CAUTION

If your partner has sensitive skin or suffers from allergies, massage with just one drop of essential oil per 20ml/4 tsp base oil at first to test for any reaction. Always seek medical advice before massaging a pregnant woman.

The oil for the massage, blended with essential oil, should be poured into a small, clean bowl from where you can take more oil from time to time without disturbing the rhythm of the massage. It is always a good idea to stand the bowl of oil on a towel in order to protect the underlying surface from spills.

MIXING OILS FOR MASSAGE

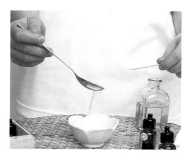

1 Pour about 10ml/2 tsp of your chosen vegetable oil into a blending bowl.

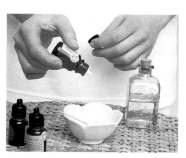

2 Add the essential oil, one drop at a time. Mix with a clean dry cocktail stick or toothpick.

Aromatherapy blends

A selection of blends of essential oils for everyday circumstances is given below. These few suggestions are to be used as a guide. If you already have a favourite blend, there is no reason why you should not use it.

Choose up to four essential oils to make an appropriate blend. Mix with a carrier or base oil.

▶ THE VARIETY OF CARRIER OILS INCLUDES ALMOND, SUNFLOWER, SESAME AND JOJOBA.

TO AID RELAXATION

For a relaxing massage choose three or four oils from the following list: bergamot, clary sage, lavender, sandalwood and German chamomile. Inlcude one of the citrus oils, to add an uplifting note to the blend.

REMEDY FOR OVER-INDULGENCE

A gentle massage using three or four of any of the following oils may help to restore balance following an over-indulgent period: orange, black pepper, geranium, juniper and ginger.

▼ CAREFULLY MEASURE OUT THE CORRECT QUANTITY OF BASE OIL.

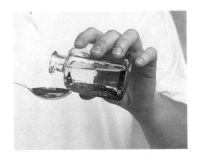

TO DISPEL GLOOM

Try making a blend of three or four of the following essential oils: black pepper, cypress, eucalyptus, ginger, grapefruit, jasmine, juniper, lemon, nutmeg, peppermint, rosemary and tea tree.

FOR STIFF MUSCLES

Everyone suffers from minor muscular aches and pains from time to time. Warming essential oils are the most helpful for stiff muscles. You can choose from any of the following: black pepper, ginger, clary sage, eucalyptus,

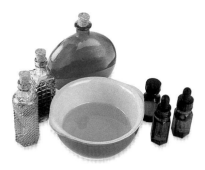

◀ Mix your blend of essential oils with a carrier, or base, oil in a small bowl ready for use.

peppermint, grapefruit, jasmine, juniper, lavender, lemon, orange, marjoram and nutmeg.

An aphrodisiac blend

Tension, anxiety, worry, depression – all these can affect your sexual energy. This can result in a downward spiral of anxiety about sex, and cause reduced enjoyment. Try to take time out of your hectic life to spend time together with your partner and have fun: add to your sensual pleasure with an intimate massage session, using one of these blends to release tensions and allow your natural sexual energy to respond.

Use a blend that appeals to you both – either five drops rose and five drops sandalwood or four drops jasmine and four drops ylang ylang and include in a massage oil. Use gentle, stroking movements all over the back, buttocks, legs and front.

Sensual massage

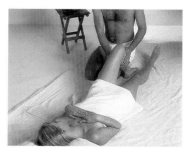

1 Use rose and sandalwood, or jasmine and ylang ylang oil to massage gently all over the body.

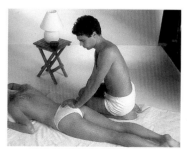

2 Apply a firmer pressure when massaging large muscles such as the buttocks.

Facial massage

A face massage dissolves anxiety and stress, eases away headaches, and enhances relaxation. Let your strokes be firm but gentle, following the natural symmetry of the bone structure and facial features.

Receiving a face massage is a wonderful way to finish a body massage, or combined with the chest, neck and head strokes, it can be a deeply satisfying and effective session in its own right.

When giving your partner a face massage, you should try to focus your total attention on to your hands and fingers so that each touch is feather like and made with great sensitivity.

GENTLE STROKES

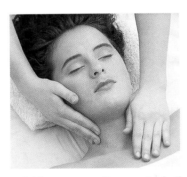

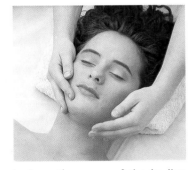

1 Add a very small amount of oil to your hands to ensure a smooth glide over the skin. Then softly stroke your hands, one following the other, up over the chest, neck and sides of the face, moulding them to the natural contours of the face.

2 A gentle caress of the jawline will be comforting to your partner. With slightly cupped hands, stroke one hand after the other in alternating movements along both sides of the face. Move from the point of the chin round towards the ears.

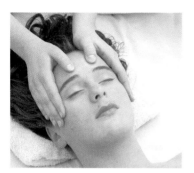

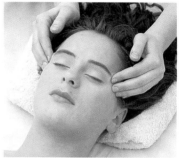

1 Place your thumbs on the forehead, while your hands cradle the face. Draw the thumbs towards the side, finishing with a sweep around the temples.

2 Keeping your hands relaxed and cupped, use your fingertips to stroke the temples very softly several times in a clockwise circular movement.

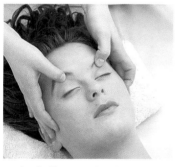

TIP
Choose the blend of oils for the massage according to your partner's needs: if they are tense and over-tired, a relaxing blend of lavender, chamomile and clary sage oils could be helpful; if they need to be revitalized, geranium and bergamot oils will give them an energizing boost.

3 The hollows under the ridge of the brow are sinus passages. Gentle pressure on these points can help to release tension headaches. Press sensitively up under the ridge, on one spot at a time, with your thumb pads.

Continue to hold the pressure under the ridge for a count of five before releasing it slowly. Move from the inner to the outer edge of the eyebrows.

facial massage **23**

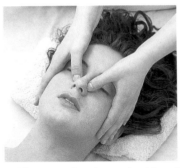

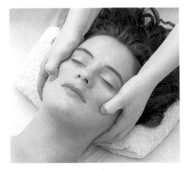

1 Slip your thumbs each side of the bridge of the nose, while wrapping your hands against the sides of the cheeks. Slide both thumbs down each side of the nose to the edge of the nostrils.

2 Without breaking the flow of motion, draw your thumb pads out under the cheekbones, indenting them slightly up under the ridge of the bone.

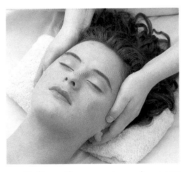

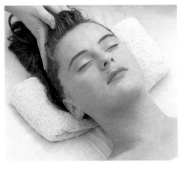

3 Soften the pressure in your thumbs as they reach the sides of the face, and begin to pull both hands soothingly up towards the top of the head.

4 Continue by drawing your hands and fingers out through the head and hair until they pull away from the body. Bring your hands back to the first position of the stroke. Repeat twice.

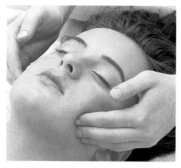

1 Relax your hands and sink your fingertips into the cheek muscles. Rotate them, counter-clockwise, several times on one area before moving to the next fleshy area.

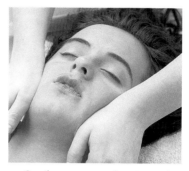

2 Gently press and rotate the heels of your hands in continuous but alternate movements on the cheeks to increase suppleness and to loosen the muscles surrounding the mouth.

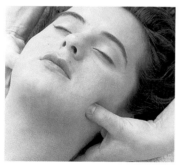

3 To reduce tension in the jaw muscles, slip your fingers behind the neck, and sink your thumbs into the muscle before rotating them on one spot at a time.

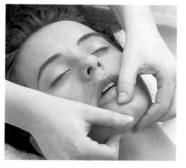

4 Grip the jaw bone with your fingers and use your thumbs to stroke over the chin in small circles, applying more pressure on the down and outward slide.

facial massage **25**

Self-massage

Give yourself a real treat with these simple self-massage techniques. Choose an appropriate blend of essential oils, and add at 1 per cent dilution to a base oil such as sweet almond. Oil your hands before spreading it on to your skin.

Self-massage is an excellent way to help yourself relax and can help clear tension headaches and ease a stiff neck and shoulders. There is an undoubted sensuality about massage, the feel of oil on the skin and the gradual easing of tension, so enjoy this opportunity to pamper yourself. The benefit is not only from the gentle application of massage oil but also from the time taken to care for yourself and your needs.

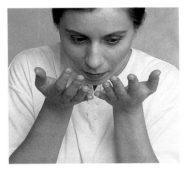

▲ Depending on the oil used, the aroma of an essential oil massage can help to relax and ease tension or uplift your mind and energize your body.

The face

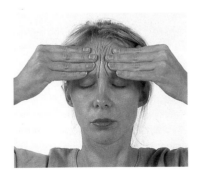

1 Use small circling movements with the fingers, over the forehead, temples and cheeks.

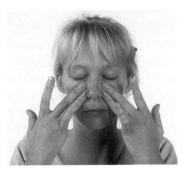

2 Work across the cheeks and along each side of the nose, then out to the jaw line.

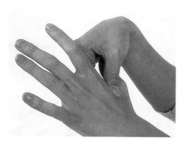

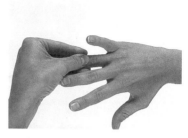

1 You can help to reduce any tension in your hands by firmly squeezing the fleshy area between each finger with the thumb and fingers of the other hand, rolling the flesh a little to give a kneading effect.

2 Squeeze and gently stretch each finger one after the other, working from the base of your finger out towards the tip. Now repeat this exercise on the other hand.

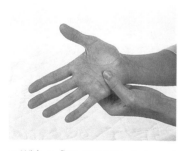

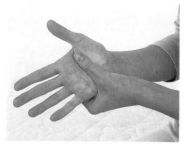

3 With a firm movement, knead the palm with the thumb of your other hand, making strong circular strokes. This squeezes and stretches taut, contracted muscles, and should be a fairly deep action.

4 Continue this kneading action as you work steadily across the palm of your hand, maintaining a firm pressure. Now repeat these movements on the other hand.

THE LEGS

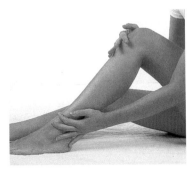

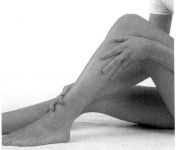

1 Sit with one leg bent, so that you can comfortably reach down as far as the ankle.

2 Sweep up the leg from ankle to knee, using alternate hands. This helps to move venous blood back towards the heart.

THE FEET

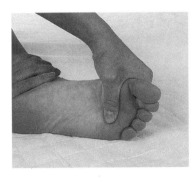

1 Sit so that you can comfortably reach a foot, and with quite a firm grip use small circular strokes all over the sole with your thumb. Pay special attention to the arch of the foot, stretching along the line of the arch with your thumb.

THE ARMS

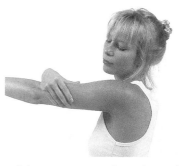 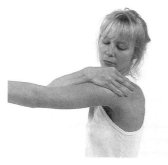

1 Grip your arm at the wrist and squeeze. Repeat this action up the length of the arm.

2 Continue up the arm to the shoulder. Switch arms and repeat the exercise.

THE SHOULDERS

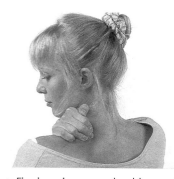 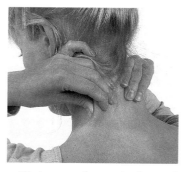

1 Firmly grip your shoulder and use a squeezing motion to loosen the tension, moving along the shoulder several times. Repeat on the other side.

2 Work up as far as the base of the skull, squeezing the neck muscles with your fingertips, and work your way down again.

Massage with a partner

One of the best ways to remove stress and tension from your partner is by massage. The effects of the following simple massage movements can be enhanced greatly by adding essential oils at 1 per cent dilution to the base oil.

When using essential oils in massage with a partner, you are sharing the therapeutic effect, so choose a blend that you both like.

Prepare the massage space beforehand so that it is warm and relaxing. Ensure that your partner is lying comfortably: use cushions or pillows for support if necessary, and cover them with towels, if needed, for warmth. Always warm the oil in your hands before applying it to the skin.

For a relaxing massage, begin with the back, move to the face, then finish with the arms and feet. This should ease headaches and tension and promote a feeling of deep and utter relaxation. Always use gentle strokes.

THE BACK

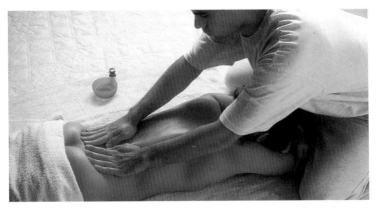

Place your hands on either side of the spine, on the line of muscles that run down the back. Move down the back using a slow gliding motion. Take your hands further out to the side and glide back up towards the shoulders, before repeating this stroke.

The face

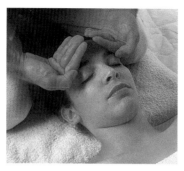

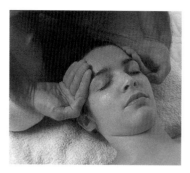

1 Smooth across the forehead with the back of your hands. Start the stroking motion at the centre of the forehead and move towards the temples.

2 These movements can often ease a headache, especially when it is still at an early stage, and are very calming.

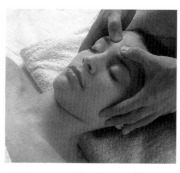

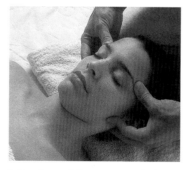

3 Using your thumbs or fingers, work steadily over the forehead in small circles, moving out over the temples to help to ease tight, tense muscles.

4 Continue this movement down the temples to the jaw line for an even greater relaxing effect. Use firm pressure, squeezing the skin with each circle.

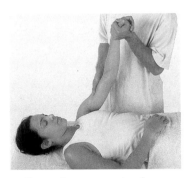

1 Support your partner's arm, raising it into the air and squeeze down the whole length of the arm with your thumb and fingers to encourage the blood and lymph to flow back towards the heart.

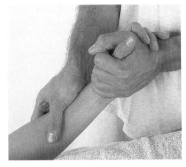

2 Let the upper arm rest on the floor, then work on the forearm with stroking movements from the wrist to the elbow – you may need to swap your hands to work around each side of the arm.

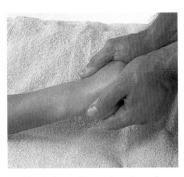

3 To help relieve tension from your partner's hands, hold one hand, palm down, in your hands and apply a steady stretching motion over the back of the hand.

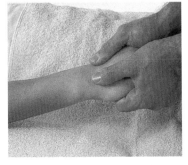

4 Repeat this stretch a few times, with a firm but comfortable pressure on the hand. Repeat all these movements on the other arm and hand.

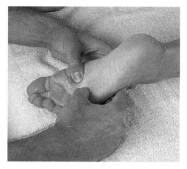

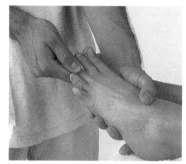

1 Use your thumbs to press firmly in small circles all over the sole. Keep the movements slow and deep, and finish with long lines running from the toes to the heel.

2 Hold one of the toes and give a squeeze and pulling action. Repeat for all the toes.

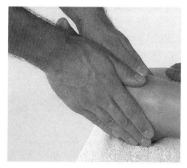

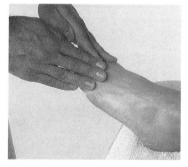

3 Smooth all the way up and down the upper side of the foot with both hands.

4 Extend the stroking from the ankle to the toes, then return to the centre; smooth back up the foot. Repeat on the other foot.

Baby massage

 All babies thrive on being cuddled, touched, and massaged. Skin-to-skin contact is essential to the nurturing of infants, helping them to bond with their parents, and to develop emotional and physical health.

SOOTHING AND FEATHERING

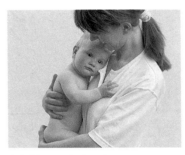

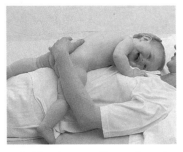

1 Hold your baby close to you, so she can feel the warmth of your body, the beat of your heart, and the rhythm of your breathing, enabling her to be comforted.

2 Babies love to lie against the softness of your body. Soothe her by placing one hand over the base of her spine, while gently stroking her head.

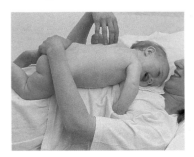

3 Running your fingertips up and down your baby's back will make her giggle as the feather-like touches brush her delicate skin.

OILS FOR BABIES AND YOUNGSTERS
Choose from the following essential oils:
Newborn infants: chamomile, geranium, lavender, mandarin and eucalyptus.
Infants 2-6 months old: as above plus neroli and peppermint.
Infants 6-12 months old: as above plus grapefruit, palmarosa and tea tree.

FLEXING AND WIGGLING

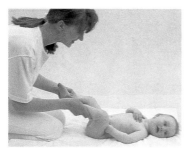

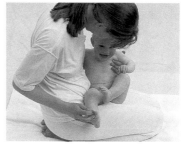

4 Your baby will enjoy this game of passive movements. Bend her knee towards her body and then straighten out her leg. Carry out the same action on the other leg. Repeat several times.

5 Babies never seem to lose interest in their fingers and toes; add to this fascination by wiggling and rotating the little joints one by one.

EFFLEURAGE

KNEADING AND SQUEEZING

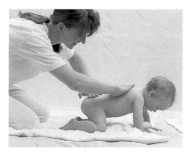

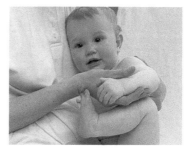

6 If your baby can keep still for long enough, you can rub nourishing oil into her skin while massaging. Soft effleurage strokes on her back, such as fanning and circles, will delight her.

7 Chubby little arms and legs are made for gentle squeezing and kneading. Press the limbs softly between your thumb and fingers.

Treatments: energizers

There are unfortunately times in all our lives when we get depressed, whether due to a specific event or from chronic tiredness. As part of a programme of recuperation and restoring vitality, aromatherapy can be very effective.

UPLIFTING OILS

For a strong, but relatively short-lived effect, try four drops bergamot and two drops neroli in the bath, ideally in the morning. After the bath, gently pat the skin with a soft towel. Do not rub vigorously. A gentler effect, which can pervade the atmosphere all day long, is to use bergamot or neroli oils in an essential oil burner – probably just one drop of each oil at a time, repeating as needed.

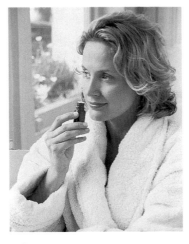

▲ ESSENTIAL OILS CAN PROVIDE AN INSTANT PICK-ME-UP.

INVIGORATING OILS

Chronic tension all too often leads to a feeling of exhaustion, when we just run out of steam. At these times we need a boost, and many oils have a tonic effect, restoring vitality without over-stimulating. As a group, citrus oils are good for this purpose, ranging from the soothing mandarin to the refreshing lemon oil.

Have a warm bath, with four drops mandarin and two drops orange or four drops neroli and two drops lemon. Alternatively, just add a couple of drops of

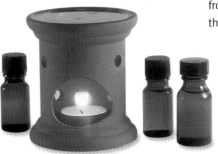

◄ VAPORIZED OILS CAN HAVE A VERY UPLIFTING EFFECT ON THE SPIRITS.

◀ LEMON OIL
REFRESHES AND
CLEARS THE MIND.

▶ ROSEMARY IS
USEFUL FOR MENTAL
FATIGUE OR LETHARGY.

any of these oils to a bowl of steaming water and gently inhale to help to lift tiredness and raise your spirits.

Steam inhalation is a valuable and simple way to receive the benefits of essential oils when time or circumstance prevents massage or a bath.

REVITALIZING OILS

In today's high pressure world, trying to juggle with too many demands leads nearly all of us to reach a state of "brain fag" at some point, when mental fatigue and exhaustion grind us to a halt.

Rather than reach for the coffee, or worse still alcohol, which may seem to relax but actually depresses the central nervous system, try using these revitalizing oils to give you an instant pick-me-up and make you feel more alert.

You can use one to two drops of rosemary or peppermint oil in a burner. Alternatively, add three drops rosemary and two drops peppermint to a bowl of steaming water, or use four drops of either oil on their own. Allow the oils to evaporate into the room.

▾ A STEAM INHALATION OF ESSENTIAL OILS
CAN HELP TO UPLIFT YOUR SPIRITS.

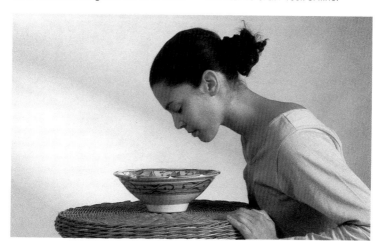

Inhalations

Colds and sinus problems may cause congestion, but we can also feel blocked up and unable to breathe freely through tension. Steam inhalations warm and moisten the membranes, and essential oils help to open the airways.

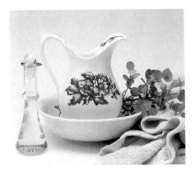

◀ A EUCALYPTUS STEAM INHALATION HELPS TO CLEAR CONGESTION.

▼ INHALE THE STEAM DEEPLY.

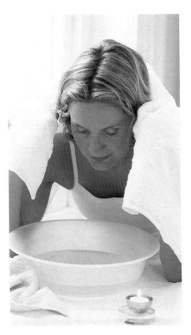

For a stuffed-up feeling, maybe combined with tiredness, try using three drops eucalyptus and two drops peppermint oil in a bowl of steaming water.

For tension causing poor breathing, relax the airways with four drops lavender and three drops frankincense.

Steam inhalations are helpful for respiratory complaints. Use a total of ten drops for a strong medicinal effect, in cases of colds and chestiness, or just five drops for a gentler relaxing effect. Inhale the steam deeply while holding a towel over your head to slow down the rate of oil evaporation.

Compresses

Hot or cold compresses are excellent ways to use oils for problems such as sprains and muscular aches. To make a compress, add essential oils to iced or hot water and soak a pad in it before placing on the affected area.

Cold compresses are suitable for use on acute injuries such as a strain or sprain, with swelling or bruising. For older injuries, for chronic muscle aches such as backache and menstrual pain, and for arthritic or rheumatic pain, a hot compress may be more useful.

The ideal oil for a cold compress is lavender, which is useful in many first-aid situations. Use four drops to a bowl of iced water. Keep the pad on for at least 20 minutes. Raise the affected limb if a swelling occurs.

For muscular aches, try using two drops of both rosemary and marjoram in a bowl of hot water. Apply for 30 minutes.

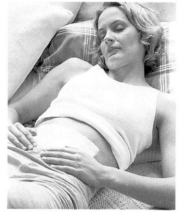

▲ USE A HOT COMPRESS TO EASE CHRONIC MENSTRUAL PAIN.

▼ A COLD COMPRESS IS GOOD FOR SOOTHING STRAINS AND SPRAINS.

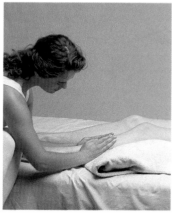

▼ COMPRESSES CAN STIMULATE CIRCULATION.

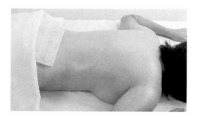

Backache relievers

So often people carry around their tensions in the form of a stiff, aching or knotted back. Symptoms can range from tight shoulders to lower backache. The best way of using oils to relieve backache is in massage of the taut muscles.

When massaging your partner's back to relieve pain, long sweeping strokes along the length of the back and a deep kneading action with the hands will loosen areas of muscle spasm, while the aromatic essential oils will work their magic and relax tension.

Two essential oil blends that will help to work on deeper tensions and knotted muscles are three drops pine and three drops rosemary oil, or four drops lavender used with three drops marjoram oil mixed with the base oil. The oil for the massage should be poured into a small, clean bowl close to hand, from where you can take more oil from time to time as you need it without disturbing the rhythm of the massage.

▸ PENETRATING ROSEMARY OIL IS PARTICULARLY BENEFICIAL FOR RELIEVING MUSCULAR ACHES.

RELAXING TENSE BACKS

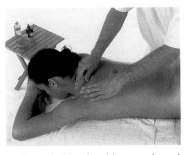

1 Knead the shoulders and neck to ease stiff, tense muscles.

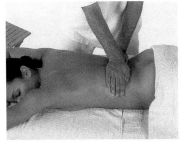

2 Apply steady, sweeping movements down the back with your hands. Finally, stroke firmly down the back with both hands.

Muscular ache relievers

When you are under stress for any length of time, your body stays permanently tense. This can make any or all of your muscles ache and feel tired or heavy. Massage with a blend of essential oils will begin to relieve symptoms.

Gentle but firm massage is a wonderful reviver of tired, tender or tense muscles, especially when the aches are smoothed away with a fragrant oil. As the massage movements start to work on the aching muscles, the oils are being absorbed and get to work on inner tension too.

For the best effect, use a blend of three drops pine, three drops marjoram and two drops juniper oil for a variety of soothing massage strokes. Other warming oils that help to relieve aching muscles include: black pepper, clary sage, eucalyptus, ginger, grapefruit, jasmine, lavender, lemon, peppermint, orange, nutmeg and rosemary. You can also try experimenting with different blends of essential oils to discover which ones suit you best.

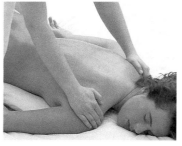

▸ A MASSAGE WITH PINE OIL IS IDEAL FOR INVIGORATING TIRED MUSCLES.

MASSAGING ACHING BACK MUSCLES

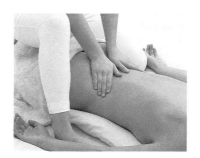

1 Rest your hands on the lower back on either side of the spine. Lean your weight into your hands and stroke firmly up the back. Mould your hands to the body as you go.

2 As your hands reach the top of your partner's back, fan them gently out towards the shoulders using a smooth, flowing motion.

Headache soothers

Tension headaches are a common feature in many people's lives, and may come from long hours at the computer or even longer hours with small children! Whatever the cause, gentle massage can help.

To relieve headaches, gentle massage of the temples and forehead at the earliest moment can help to stop headaches from getting a tight grip. Another option is the application of a warm compress soaked in hot water blended with essential oils.

If your head feels hot, try using an oil with four drops of peppermint. If warmth feels helpful, then you could try applying six drops of lavender oil. Another option for soothing a headache caused by congestion or tension is to use four drops of chamomile oil.

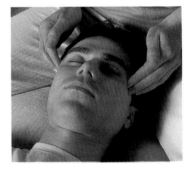

▲ PEPPERMINT

RELIEVING A HEADACHE

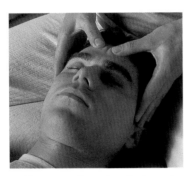

1 Ease tension headaches by massaging aromatherapy oils into the forehead. With your thumbs, use steady but gentle pressure to stroke the forehead.

2 Gently massage the temples with your fingers, using slow rotating movements, in order to ease aches and pains caused by too much stress and tension.

◀ MARJORAM

▶ CLARY SAGE

One of the most complex of health problems, migraines are nature's way of shutting our systems down when life has been too demanding. The triggers that spark off a migraine attack are highly individual and professional treatment is really needed to try to understand the causes for each person.

At the first sign of a migraine, try using a blend of two drops rosemary, one drop marjoram and one drop clary sage, diluted in a base oil and gently massaged into the forehead and temples. Alternatively, use a drop of each essential oil in a bowl of warm water and apply a warm compress to the forehead.

ALLEVIATING A MIGRAINE

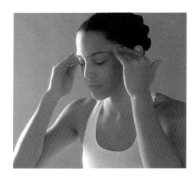

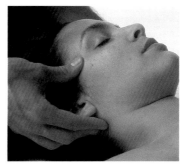

1 Many migraine sufferers have a heightened sense of smell at the onset of the attack and may find any aroma intolerable, so use oils sparingly. For self-help, gently massage the temples with small circling movements.

2 Receiving a gentle head massage from a partner allows you to lie back and relax your body completely and can therefore be even more effective than a self-massage at soothing the pain.

Menstrual pain easers

Painful periods can be due to several factors, but tension will certainly add to muscle spasm and cramping pains. If there is no organic or structural cause of the discomfort, try using essential oils as a hot compress or in the bath.

Some essential oils have a reputation for improving the menstrual cycle in ways other than as a compress or added to a hot bath; seek advice from a professional aromatherapist for longer-term treatments.

For a hot compress, soak a pad in hot water mixed with one drop each of rose, geranium and clary sage essential oils. Apply the compress over the lower abdomen to relieve menstrual pain. Alternatively, a fairly hot bath with three drops of rose, three drops of geranium and two drops of clary sage oil will quickly relax the cramped or aching muscles.

▲ Rose

▼ A HOT BATH WITH OILS IS RELAXING.

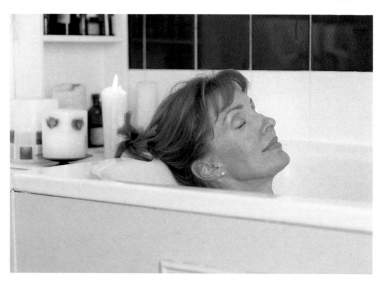

For many women the days leading up to a period can be fraught with mood swings, irritability and other symptoms. Professional treatment may be needed for full assistance; however, you could try this blend of essential oils if before each period you feel very tense and critical of those around you, or you just want to devour a box of chocolates!

Add three drops rose, three drops jasmine and two drops

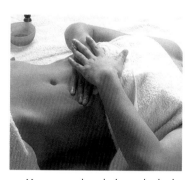

▶ JASMINE

clary sage essential oil to a hot bath and lie back, allowing the aroma to soothe you, and the warm water to soak away any tension in your body. Alternatively, you could try using this mixture in a massage oil and rub it gently into your lower abdomen for a soothing and relaxing effect.

PREMENSTRUAL TENSION SOOTHER

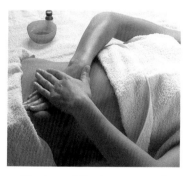

1 Slowly and firmly massage the lower abdomen with your hands. Close your eyes and continue the massage until you feel relaxed.

2 Move your hands in a clockwise direction, working upwards towards the chest; try to remain relaxed the whole time so that the tension drains away.

Digestive settlers

Nervousness often results in an upset stomach. It has been said that our digestive organs also digest stress, and can end up storing emotions, causing discomfort and indigestion. The key is to let our bodies release anxieties.

Aromatherapy can help a great deal to achieve relaxation and calmness, allowing our bodies to release stress which may affect the digestive organs. One of the easiest ways to use oils in this context is to make a hot compress and place it over the abdomen, keeping the area warm for up to ten minutes.

To make the hot compress, add to a bowl of hot water either two drops orange and three drops peppermint oil or three drops chamomile and two drops orange essential oils. Soak a flannel in the scented water, wring it out, and apply it over the abdomen as directed above. The heat from the compress will soothe away stress and tension, and relax the abdominal muscles. Use the compress as often as necessary for relief, ensuring the flannel remains hot.

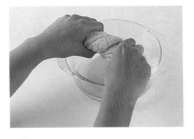

▲ SOAK A FLANNEL IN HOT WATER.

▼ LAY THE COMPRESS OVER THE ABDOMEN.

▼ SOOTHING PEPPERMINT TEA.

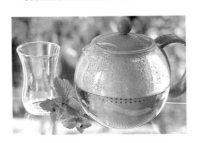

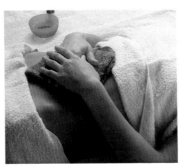

Travel calmers

It is said that travel broadens the mind; unfortunately, for some people it contracts the mind into a series of worries. Is this plane safe? Will I be sick? Try one of the following essential oils to calm the mind and stomach.

Inhaling essential oils while travelling allows you to enjoy the anticipation of new horizons without being stressed by how to reach them. The simplest way for you to use essential oils when travelling is to put a couple of drops onto a tissue or handkerchief, and to inhale them frequently. Useful aromatherapy oils for

◀ PEPPERMINT

▶ MANDARINS

this purpose include peppermint, mandarin and neroli. In addition to helping overcome travel sickness, peppermint is also useful for muscular aches and pains, nausea and colds. Mandarin oil has an uplifting effect and is also a good oil to use for treating restlessness and nervous tension. Likewise, neroli oil is useful during times of anxiety.

CALMING OILS

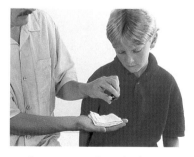

1 Put a couple of drops of aromatherapy oil onto a tissue or folded handkerchief.

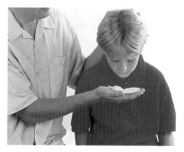

2 Hold the tissue under the nose and lean the head slightly forwards. Inhale. Repeat as necessary throughout the journey.

Hair care

These days there is a bewildering range of products available for every type of hair. However, simpler treatments, which have been tried and trusted over many years, can also make your hair look wonderful.

Good hairdressers recommend a varied programme of hair care because consistently using one product can lead to build-up on the hair and scalp. Herbal hair rinses, shampoos and other treatments use natural ingredients which will leave your hair in really good condition.

The easiest way to make a herbal shampoo is to add 30–45ml/2-3 tbsp of a strong herbal infusion to a baby shampoo. Alternatively, you could

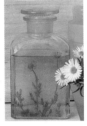

▸ STORE HERBAL HAIR RINSES IN GLASS BOTTLES.

add two to three drops of your favourite oil. For chamomile and orangeflower shampoo, mix 15ml/1 tbsp chamomile infusion and five drops neroli essential oil into 60ml/4 tbsp mild shampoo just before washing your hair.

HERBAL RINSE

A herbal rinse helps to keep the hair shiny and in good condition. When washing your hair, simply replace the last water rinse with a jugful of herbal rinse, mixed with water 50/50, and leave to dry. Chamomile and rosemary have been combined with vinegar and used in hair rinses for hundreds of years. The herbs enhance the colour of the hair and the vinegar is a wonderful scalp conditioner.

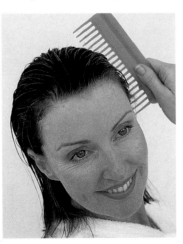

◂ COMB HAIR TREATMENT THROUGH HAIR.

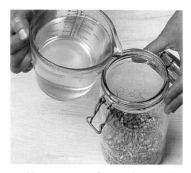

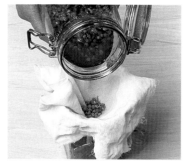

1 Measure 50g/2oz chamomile flowers in a jar. Pour 900ml/ 1½ pints boiled water over them.

2 Seal the jar and leave to stand overnight. Strain through muslin until the mixture is clear.

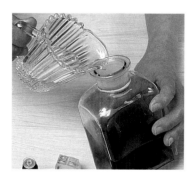

3 Add 50ml/2fl oz cider vinegar and five drops of chamomile essential oil. Store the mixture in a stoppered glass bottle in the fridge and use, within one week, as a final rinse whenever you wash your hair. The chamomile will enhance your hair's natural colour without bleaching.

DARK-HAIR RINSE

This rinse uses the same basic ingredients as the fair-hair rinse but substitutes sprigs of fresh rosemary and rosemary oil for the chamomile flowers and oil. Pregnant women, however, should omit the rosemary essential oil.

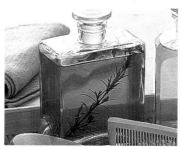

Skin care

When we become stressed, the small muscles close to the skin tend to contract. This can leave our skin under-nourished with blood, and our complexion and skin tone suffer. Using essential oils can help counteract this.

Tense skin is frequently much drier than normal skin, and probably the best way to use essential oils is to mix them into your favourite skin cream. Obviously, this is best if the skin cream is originally unperfumed.

To make a reviving skin tonic, add three drops sandalwood and three drops rose oil, or four drops neroli and two drops rose oil to a 25g/1oz pot of skin cream. Mix together and apply to the skin.

To make a fragrant rose lotion which is excellent for all skin types, mix 175ml/6fl oz unscented

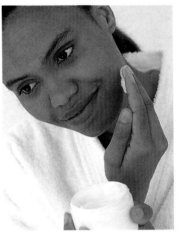

▲ APPLYING OIL-BLENDED SKIN CREAM.

body lotion with ten drops rose essential oil. Pour into a bottle with a tight lid to store. A refreshing, lightly fragranced citrus body lotion can be made in the same way using 175ml/6fl oz unscented body lotion, ten drops grapefruit essential oil and five drops bergamot essential oil; however, do not apply this lotion before going into the sun.

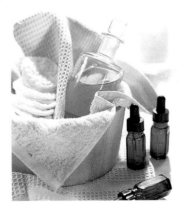

◀ OIL-SCENTED BODY LOTION IS BEST APPLIED AFTER A WARM BATH.

▶ IT IS BEST IF YOU ONLY MIX UP SMALL AMOUNTS OF CREAM AND OIL AT A TIME.

CLASSIC CLEANSERS

Gentle but effective cleansers are easy to make from pure, simple ingredients. Soapwort cleansing liquid is made by placing 15g/½ oz chopped soapwort root (available from herbalists) in a pan with 600ml/1 pint bottled spring water. Bring to the boil and simmer for 15 minutes. Strain the infusion through a paper filter, then stir in 50ml/2fl oz rose water and decant the mixture into a glass bottle. This will keep for a month in the fridge.

Another classic cleanser is almond oil cleanser, which is a traditional mix of beeswax,

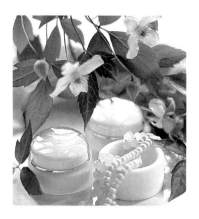

almond oil and rose water. Melt 25g/1oz white beeswax in a double boiler and whisk in 150ml/5fl oz almond oil. In a pan, add 1.5ml/¼ tsp borax (available from chemists) to 60ml/4 tbsp rose water and warm gently to dissolve. Slowly add the rose water mixture to the oils, whisking all the time. Add a few drops of rose essential oil. Continue to whisk until the mixture has a smooth, creamy texture. Pour the cleanser into a container and leave to cool. Replace the lid. To use the cleanser, smooth it on to the skin using a circular movement and remove with damp cotton wool.

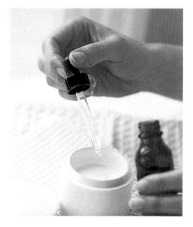

◀ ADDING DROPS OF OIL TO SKIN CREAM.

Hand care

Our hands frequently suffer from poor circulation and damage caused from overuse and abuse. Warm hand baths and the application of hand cream relieve poor circulation, soothe the skin and heal any cuts.

HAND BATHS

Circulation to our extremities is affected by tension and stress, among other things. The warmth of the water in a hand bath can help the blood vessels to dilate, which can be helpful in treating tension headaches and migraines, when the blood vessels in the head are frequently engorged with blood. If you regularly suffer from these problems, try a hand bath at the first signs of a headache to drain away the excess stress.

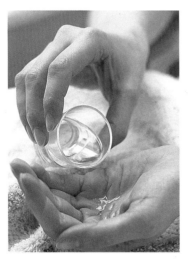

▲ RELAX TIRED HANDS WITH A BLEND OF ROSEMARY AND PINE ESSENTIAL OILS.

▼ A WARM HAND BATH CAN HELP TO RELIEVE POOR CIRCULATION IN THE HANDS.

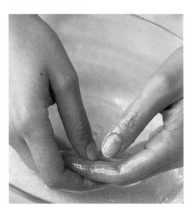

For poor circulation and tense, cold fingers, add two drops lavender and two drops marjoram essential oils to a large bowl two-thirds filled with hot water. Soak your hands in the bowl of water for relief of discomfort.

To relieve over-exertion causing tension and stiffness, try a blend of two drops rosemary and two drops pine in a bowl of hot water.

Hand creams

You can make hand creams by adding suitable essential oils to an unscented cream. Look for a lanolin-rich cream or one that includes cocoa butter as hands benefit from a richer formulation. For a healing cream (see below) blend chamomile, geranium and lemon with unscented hand cream. Store the cream in a plastic bottle.

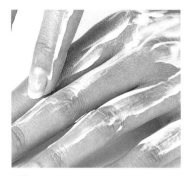

▲ You should always try to remember to moisturize your hands at least twice a day.

Preparing a healing hand cream

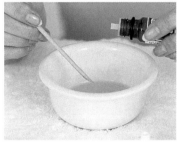

1 Blend ten drops chamomile with five drops geranium and lemon.

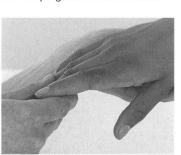

2 Blend the oils with 120ml/4fl oz unscented hand cream.

3 Spread the hand cream over the hands and rub it in thoroughly. The cream is healing because the chamomile oil soothes rough skin, the geranium oil helps heal cuts and the lemon oil softens the skin.

Foot care

Feet often suffer from neglect. We take them for granted, and seldom care for them the way we do the rest of the body. Warming foot baths and soothing foot creams are two ways of relieving neglected feet.

FOOT BATHS

Just as hands can be treated with a warm hand bath, feet can also benefit from a foot bath to which has been added three or four drops of essential oil. The warmth of the water helps circulation to improve and soothes aches and pains.

Peppermint essential oil is cooling, counteracts tiredness and is the ideal oil for using in a refreshing foot bath. For hot, aching feet, add two drops peppermint and two drops lemon oil to a large bowl two-thirds filled with hot water. Soak your feet in the water for instant relief.

If you suffer from poor circulation in your toes, add two drops lavender and two drops marjoram oil to a bowl of hot water. Soak your feet until warmed through.

▼ RELAX WITH A WARM FOOT BATH.

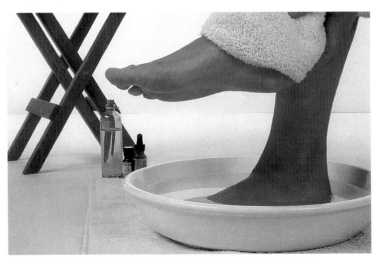

▶ MOISTURIZE YOUR FEET WITH A SOOTHING FOOT CREAM BLENDED WITH ESSENTIAL OILS.

FOOT CREAMS

You can easily make your own foot cream by adding suitable essential oils to an unscented cream. Tea tree is one of the best essential oils to incorporate in a foot cream. It has healing, antiseptic properties as well as a fungicidal action, which will protect the feet from the various foot complaints that can be picked up at the pool or gym.

To prepare tea tree foot cream, blend 15 drops tea tree essential oil thoroughly into 120ml/4fl oz unscented lanolin-rich cream (or one that includes cocoa butter). Pour the blended cream into a plastic storage bottle using a

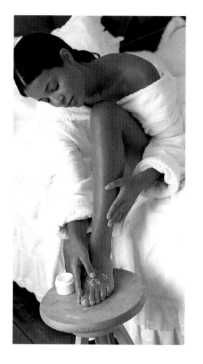

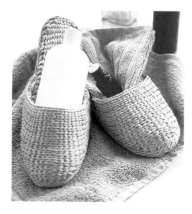

funnel. Although most creams and lotions are best stored in glass or ceramic containers, it is more practical to keep the foot cream in a pump-action plastic bottle.

To use the foot cream, simply press the plunger to release a small amount of cream on to your hands, and rub all over your feet to soothe and heal. Apply as often as required.

◀ SET ASIDE TIME TO PAMPER YOUR FEET.

Bathing

Imagine soaking in a hot bath, enveloped in a delicious scent of exotic flowers, feeling all the day's tensions drop away . . . well, it can be a reality with aromatherapy. The scented essential oils immediately soothe and relax.

Essential oils make a luxurious addition to the bath, whether they are chosen to aid recovery from a particular illness, to lift the spirits, or to promote relaxation after a stressful day. The essential oils that are recommended for the bath affect the body as they are

▶ USE ESSENTIAL OIL BURNERS TO ADD THERAPEUTIC SCENTS TO YOUR ROOMS.

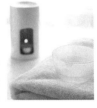

inhaled in the steam, but some will also cling to the skin and penetrate through skin pores that have opened in the warm atmosphere. In order to add the oils to the bath safely it is important to dilute them. There are a variety of ways to do this, the most common of which is to use a vegetable oil – any one of the carrier oils used for massage will be suitable. For those who do not need or like an oily bath, a commercial dispersing agent (available from health food shops), some ordinary dairy cream, or full-fat milk can be used instead. These non-slip carriers are especially important in baths for the elderly and young children.

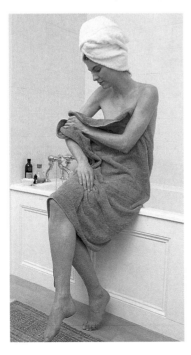

◀ GENTLY PAT YOUR SKIN DRY AFTER A BATH.

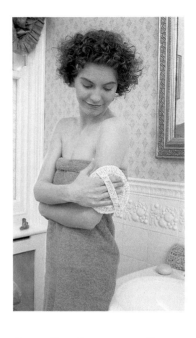

ylang ylang essential oils to add to your bath. For tired, tense and aching muscles, try soaking in a bath to which you have added three drops marjoram and two drops chamomile essential oils.

Add the blend to the water just before the bath has filled to the desired depth, pouring it in slowly under the hot water tap so that the oil is dispersed through the air and the water. After the bath, gently pat the skin dry with a soft towel. Avoid a vigorous rub-down.

Preparation for an aromatherapy bath should include the removal of dead skin cells. Use a massage mitt or a thoroughly dampened loofah, and rub it firmly but gently over the whole body.

SUGGESTED OIL BLENDS

For a refreshing, uplifting bath in the mornings try a blend of three drops bergamot and two drops geranium essential oils.

To relax and unwind after a long day, make a blend of three drops lavender and two drops

▼ CANDLES CREATE A SENSUAL ATMOSPHERE.

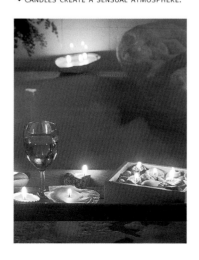

bathing **57**

De-stressers

Stress, or rather our inability to cope with an excess amount of it, is one of the biggest health problems today. Regardless of how we react to stress, we can all benefit from the wonderfully balancing effects of aromatic oils.

Our bodies are geared to cope with a stressful situation by producing various hormones that trigger off a series of physiological actions in the body; these are known as the "fight or flight" syndrome, and serve to place the body in a state of alert in a potentially dangerous situation. Extra blood is shunted to the muscles, and the heart rate speeds up while the digestion slows down. These responses are appropriate when we are faced with a physical threat, but can be triggered by quite different kinds of stress and place a strain on our bodies without fulfilling any useful need. In order to help reduce the impact of stress on the whole system, it is necessary to find ways both to avoid getting over-stressed in the first instance and to let go of the changes that occur internally under stress. Aromatherapy can help in each case, the oils helping to keep you calm under pressure and releasing inner tensions following stress, especially in massage. To prevent undue stress, you can try simply inhaling your favourite essential oil at regular intervals throughout the day.

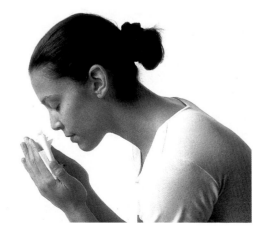

▶ INHALE ESSENTIAL OIL TO RELEASE TENSION.

If possible, use one of the following blends of essential oil in a base oil, and get your partner to massage you, for the perfect antidote to life's stresses. For aiding relaxation, use three drops lavender, three drops geranium and three drops marjoram oils. For calming and soothing, as well as giving a gentle uplift, use four drops rose and three drops jasmine oils. For a more definitely uplifting and energizing effect, try three drops clary sage and four drops bergamot essential oils.

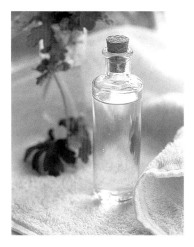

▲ GERANIUM OIL COMBINED WITH LAVENDER AND MARJORAM OILS AIDS RELAXATION.

STRESS-RELIEVING MASSAGE

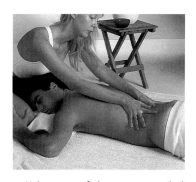

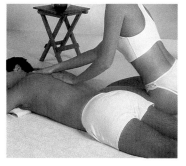

1 Using one of the recommended blends of essential oils, slowly and gently massage the oil into your partner's skin, moving your hands down each side of the spine.

2 For relaxation, use one hand after the other to stroke down the back in a steady rhythm. Continue stroking for several minutes to allow the tension to drain away.

Relaxers

When people are described as being "uptight", that is often exactly what they are: tense muscles in the face and neck are a sure sign of anxiety. Release that tension with a face massage using gently soothing strokes.

A face massage using soothing strokes with the fingertips, on the temples and forehead especially, is very good as an evening treat, calming away the day's cares and relaxing tense muscles. Use just a little oil, as most people dislike a greasy feeling on the face. Make up a blend of four drops lavender and two drops ylang ylang oils in a light oil such as sweet almond, grapeseed or coconut.

▸ THE SCENT OF LAVENDER HELPS THE BODY AND MIND TO UNWIND.

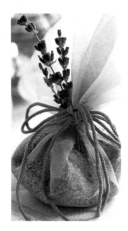

SMOOTHING AWAY TENSION

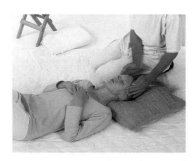

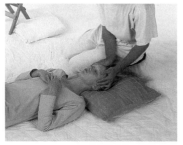

1 Have the person lying down with the head on a cushion or in your lap. With your fingertips, gently smooth the essential oil blend into the face and head.

2 Using your thumbs one after the other, stroke tension away from the centre of the forehead.

Sleep inducers

Worries can race around inside our heads, usually just as we are trying to fall asleep. The resulting restless night leaves us prone to anxiety. Help break this cycle with a hot, relaxing evening bath using essential oils.

Many essential oils can be added to a bath to aid relaxation and sleep. Just having a fragrance that you enjoy will help you to unwind after a long day.

A couple of relaxing blends, which are not over-sedating, are three drops sandalwood oil and four drops rose, or five drops lavender and three drops ylang ylang oil. Add the oils to the bath just before you get in, holding them under the hot water tap so they are dispersed evenly in the air and water.

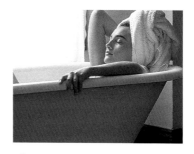

▲ UNWIND IN A FRAGRANT BATH.

Other essential oils that aid relaxation include bergamot, chamomile and clary sage, while tranquillity and peacefulness can be achieved with neroli.

▼ MAKE AROMATHERAPY PART OF YOUR BATHING ROUTINE.

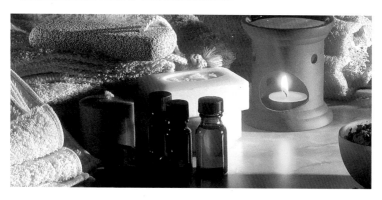

Properties of essential oils

This chart provides a ready reference to those essential oils that are suitable for use in the home, together with some of the more common complaints and disorders they may be used to treat.

	ACHE	ARTHRITIS	ATHLETE'S FOOT	BAD BREATH	BOILS, BLISTERS	BRITTLE NAILS	BROKEN VEINS	BRONCHITIS, CHEST INFECTIONS	BRUISES	BURNS	CHILBLAINS	COLD SORES	CYSTITIS, URINARY INFECTIONS	DANDRUFF	DERMATITIS	EARACHE	ECZEMA
BENZOIN		•						•		•			•				
BERGAMOT	•			•				•				•	•				•
BLACK PEPPER		•															
CEDARWOOD	•	•						•					•				
CHAMOMILE	•	•			•				•	•	•		•	•		•	
CLARY SAGE	•													•			
CYPRESS								•					•				
EUCALYPTUS		•						•									
FENNEL								•									
FRANKINCENSE								•					•				
GERANIUM	•								•	•	•		•		•		•
GINGER		•															
GRAPEFRUIT	•																
JASMINE																	
JUNIPER	•	•												•	•		•
LAVENDER									•	•						•	
LEMON	•	•			•	•		•	•		•	•					
MANDARIN	•																
MARJORAM		•							•	•		•					
NEROLI							•	•									
NUTMEG		•															
ORANGE								•									
PALMAROSA	•													•	•		
PEPPERMINT	•			•				•							•		
ROSE							•									•	
ROSEMARY	•							•						•	•	•	
ROSEWOOD	•														•		
SANDALWOOD	•							•					•				•
TEA TREE	•		•					•		•		•	•	•		•	
YLANG YLANG																	

FLU	HEAVY PERIODS	HICCUPS	INSECT BITES	IRREGULAR PERIODS	LACK OF PERIODS	MENOPAUSE	MOUTH ULCERS	NEURALGIA	NOSE BLEEDS	PALPITATIONS	PERIOD PAIN	PILES (HAEMORRHOIDS)	PMS	RASHES, ALLERGIES	RHEUMATISM	SCARS	SKIN ULCERS	SORE THROATS	SPOTS	SPRAINS, STRAINS	THRUSH	WARTS, VERRUCAS	WOUNDS, CUTS, SORES
•							•						•	•				•					•
•			•															•	•			•	•
•									•						•								
															•								
	•		•			•							•	•	•					•	•		
					•		•						•	•				•					
•	•					•							•	•									
•			•																				
		•			•		•	•					•		•								
•	•													•	•	•	•	•				•	•
					•		•								•	•							•
•					•										•			•		•			
•												•											
					•						•		•					•		•			
•					•						•	•			•								•
•			•		•						•				•								•
•			•					•		•			•	•	•			•	•		•	•	
	•																		•				
					•						•		•	•					•				
•							•	•		•					•								
															•								
•							•																
											•				•							•	•
•											•												
				•							•	•			•								
•			•								•	•			•								
																		•					•
																		•					•
•			•				•						•					•	•		•	•	•
											•												

properties of essential oils **63**

index

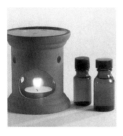

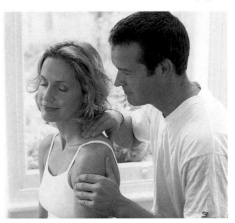